INTERMI
FOR WC

A Complete guide for women to learn what happens after they turn 60, Why They Should Go For Intermittent Fasting, Types of Intermittent Fasting with Delicious recipes to Make their Fasting Easy

By
MELINDA FRANCIS

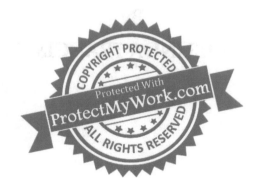

Contents

Introduction

The golden decade is a wonderful moment for a woman. They accept themselves completely and attempt to live a happy and peaceful life. Wouldn't it be wonderful if that was the case all of the time? Unfortunately, it isn't, and although women may have a good life beyond 60, several problems can put a stop to their lifestyle. As women age, their body form naturally changes. They typically start to put on weight once they hit the age of 60. Weight loss tends to happen later in life, partially due to fat replacing lean muscle tissues. A good diet can play a major impact in a woman's body transition in their life.

Women over the age of 60 may encounter difficulties when attempting to lose weight. Often, the primary factor is a slowed metabolism. A women's metabolism will be faster if they have more lean muscle. Women can influence the aging process rate by altering their ways of life. One of the things to do to slow down the aging process in the body includes Intermittent fasting (IF).

Intermittent fasting has attracted increasing attention in recent years due to the variety of health benefits it provides and the fact that it does not limit food choices. Intermittent fasting helps improve metabolism and mental wellbeing and may even help prevent certain cancers. It can also help women over 60 avoid specific nerve, muscle, and joint disorders. It is not a diet but rather a way of life. This diet will help you eat fewer calories on a daily basis and will assist you in going on with your weight loss journey. Certain women practicing IF opt for alternate-day fasting in, which they normally eat on alternate days and consume only 25% of their usual daily calorie intake on the remaining days. Others prefer their eating patterns according to the hours of the day.

Intermittent fasting has plenty of other benefits for women in their 60s. Intermittent fasting also helps lower insulin resistance, resulting in a 20-30% reduction in blood sugar and fasting insulin levels, potentially protecting from type 2 diabetes, especially in women over 60. Several studies indicate that IF reduces inflammatory indicators, which are a major contributor to the development of many chronic illnesses. Intermittent fasting also reduces cholesterol, which contributes to heart disease.

Apart from physical benefits, IF promotes a healthier mentality. It stimulates brain chemicals that help create new brain cells that combat Alzheimer's disease and promote clarity of thought for women. Intermittent fasting is a perfect way for a woman to start their 60s and feel confident like never before.

Chapter 1: What Happens To A Women's Body After 60

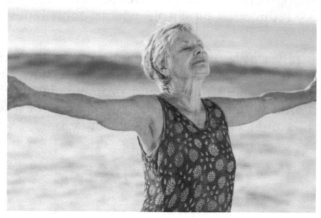

As women age, their bodies undergo changes, which are not always harmful - they are just different. Learning what to expect will assist in accepting these changes and understanding what to do to smooth the transition. While some of these transformations are imperceptible and occur gradually, others tend to happen rapidly. Whatever time they occur; it is important to understand that they are natural.

1.1 Metabolism System of Women over 60

Over the age of 60, one encounters difficulties while attempting to reduce weight. This is a major problem among women. It might be a result of a variety of factors. Often, the core problem is decreased metabolism. Metabolic rate begins to decline in women at the age of 60s after a rapid rise in teens and early twenties before ultimately leveling out in fifties.

Over the age of 60, metabolism slows down. Metabolism can get better by gaining more lean muscle. However, as women age, they drop lean muscle mass and frequently are much less active than they once were. As a result, Stubborn body fat that simply would not leave occurs.

To get rid of this problem, fasting has been shown to boost metabolism and emotional health and help avoid some malignancies.

A slowed metabolism can be caused by various factors, including

- Consuming excessive fat, which the body attempts to store by lowering the metabolic system.

- Consuming insufficient calories causes a woman's body to slow down since it assumes that the person is starving.

- A lack of physical activity might result in abdominal fat.

- Certain medicines, such as steroids, diabetic medications, and antidepressants, can cause slowed metabolism in women.

- Medical issues such as thyroid that are no longer functioning or the insulin that is no longer usable.

Any of these may be contributing factors to slowed metabolism, which might result in surprising weight gain in the long run.

1.2 HGH Production Level in Women

A crucial factor in reducing the aging process is the human growth hormone (HGH). A women's body in the 60 produces less testosterone, estrogen, and human growth hormone (HGH), which results in muscle loss - and muscle is a critical component of a healthy metabolism. A recent study has proven that HGH has a direct favorable effect on various biological functions. The pituitary gland secretes HGH during sleep and has a role in tissue healing, cell replication, and bone health. However, by the time women reach their sixties, their overall HGH levels will be around half of what they were at twenty.

As a result of the decreased HGH production, you will have

significantly decreased endurance, more body fat, a longer healing period, and a compromised immune system.

Although HGH production declines with age, some beneficial lifestyle modifications might help naturally increase HGH production for women over 60's.

The most prevalent signs of adult growth hormone insufficiency in women over 60's are as follows:

- Metabolic abnormalities in the central region (belly fat)
- Depression
- Decreased Mineral Density of the Bone
- Muscle mass loss
- Anxiety
- Insulin sensitivity is decreased
- Hypercholesterolemia
- Dysfunction of the neuromuscular system
- Decreased strength
- Muscle mass loss

Additionally, genetics may have a role in developing a deficiency. On the other hand, a significant proportion of female hormone deficiency is caused by a pituitary adenoma or its therapy (surgery, radiation, etc.). Over the last several decades, it has been shown that HGH shortage is also caused by women participating in contact sports such as basketball, rugby and boxing, and other activities that can result in traumatic brain damage and head trauma, resulting in adult GHD.

According to studies, fasting results in a significant boost in HGH levels of women over 60. One researcher discovered that HGH levels jump by more than 300 percent three days into a fast,

grown by a staggering 1,250 percent after a week of fasting. Other studies have discovered comparable results, with HGH levels doubling or tripling after only 2–3 days of fasting. On the other hand, continuous fasting is not sustainable in the long run. Intermittent fasting is an increasingly prevalent dietary strategy that restricts eating to small time intervals.

There are several techniques of intermittent fasting. A frequent technique is to alternate a daily eight-hour eating window with a sixteen-hour fast. Another includes consuming 500–600 calories twice a week. Intermittent fasting can aid in the optimization of HGH levels in two ways. To begin, it can assist in losing body fat, which has a direct effect on HGH production. Secondly, insulin is released while eating, which will keep insulin levels low for most of the day. Insulin surges may disrupt the body's natural growth hormone production. Significant changes in HGH levels occur between fasting and feeding days. 12–16-hour fasts are likely beneficial for HGH production.

1.3 Other Effects of Aging:

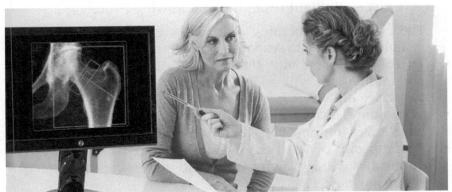

Cardiovascular System

As women grow old, their heart and blood arteries grow stiffer, and the heart fills with blood at a slower rate than it did previously. Women over 60's are more likely than younger women to acquire high blood pressure because the stiffer the

blood vessels are, the less room there is for blood vessels to expand as blood is pushed through them.

A typical older heart is still functional, but it cannot pump as much blood as a younger heart or accelerate as rapidly as a younger heart. Changes in the heart and blood arteries may occur as women age.

For example, as women become older, their heart can't beat as quickly as it could when they were younger during physical exercise or times of stress.

However, with normal aging, the number of heart beats per minute (heart rate) does not alter dramatically. Because of all of the medical advancements that have occurred in the previous two decades, the number of deaths from heart-related disorders has decreased significantly.

As women age, the heart and arteries become stiffer, making it even more crucial to do everything they can to maintain their cardiovascular system as healthy as possible. Physical exercise, such as any form of aerobic activity and a good diet, are excellent strategies.

Immune System

By reaching the decade, the immune system begins to function less effectively. It might result in the following issues:

- The chance of becoming sick increases due to the immune system's tendency to respond more slowly to stimuli.
- There is a possibility that vaccines such as the flu and pneumonia jabs will no longer be effective or last as long as they once did.
- With aging, a women's body recovers more slowly since they have fewer immune cells to fight off infection.
- The capacity of the body to identify and fix flaws in cells diminishes while growing older and increasing the chance of acquiring cancer.
- Women can develop an autoimmune illness, a condition in which the immune system targets and kills healthy bodily tissue by mistake.

It is essential to take good care to ensure that the immune system is as healthy as possible.

Receiving the vaccinations the doctor recommends, such as those for the flu (get a high-dose flu vaccine if 60 or older), pneumococcal disease, pneumonia, and shingles. Eating a proper diet, exercising regularly, abstaining from smoking, and limiting your alcohol use will help maintain the immune system in good shape.

Declining Bone Mass

Aging is caused by a variety of functional changes that result in a significant loss in all human capacities.

With aging, a range of anatomical and functional changes occur. Declining bone mass is a common concern among women over the age of 60. A woman's bones begin to lose protein matrix tissue after she has gone through menopause, resulting in increased deformation of the bones. Bone mass reaches its maximum at the age of 35 and then begins to decline as levels of estrogen decline. Women often break bones in accidents when they are in their 60s, resulting in a huge bruise, while this would have hardly affected them in their 30s.

Chapter 2: What Is Intermittent Fasting?

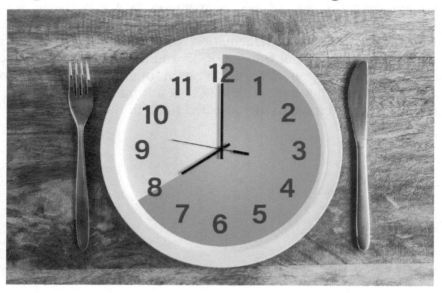

Intermittent fasting has become a popular weight-loss approach; it is not a new phenomenon. Apart from religious and spiritual motives, fasting has been practiced by numerous civilizations throughout history to improve physical and mental health. The ancient Greek athletes, for example, would fast to prepare themselves for competition in the Olympic games. But what precisely is intermittent fasting, and how does it differ from regular fasting? And more importantly, can restricting food consumption to particular intervals of the day or certain days of a week truly help lose weight?

Following is the answer to these questions. Intermittent fasting (IF) is a diet that sticks to a schedule that alternates between eating times and intervals of not eating. It is an eating approach that does not place restrictions on what one eats but on when one consumes it.

Intermittent fasting for weight reduction has been shown to enhance metabolic health and reduce insulin levels in women, allowing the body to burn more calories throughout the day.

Many different techniques for intermittent fasting exist; however, all of them revolve around alternating times of eating with periods of fasting. Choosing to eat at specific times of the day or on particular days of the week is permissible as long as the routine is consistent. Unlike other diets, which instruct on what to eat, intermittent fasting instructs when to eat by introducing frequent short-term fasts into the routine. A low-calorie diet may help lose weight while also lowering the chances of developing diabetes and heart disease. Unlike other diets, intermittent fasting does not keep track of the calories or macronutrient consumption.

There are no restrictions on which foods must be consumed or avoided, making it more like a lifestyle than a diet. Many individuals utilize intermittent fasting to lose weight because it is an easy, practical, and successful strategy to consume less and shed body fat while maintaining energy levels. It also aids in the prevention of heart diseases and diabetes, the preservation of muscular mass, and the improvement of psychological well-being. Furthermore, it has fewer meals to plan, prepare, and cook. This eating pattern might help save time in the kitchen.

2.1 Benefits of Intermittent Fasting for Women over 60's

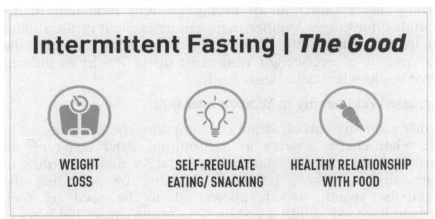

The benefits of intermittent fasting are not just derived from eating less (although this may occur when limiting the window of food availability) but also from metabolic changes that occur when spending long periods without eating.

The word autophagy is used to describe the fundamental adaption that occurs during a fast. Autophagy is the body's self-cleansing function, which activates when nutrients are insufficiently accessible to the cells. It is necessary to clear away damaged or old cells to create a place for better cells to maintain cellular and metabolic health.

Autophagy has been linked to the avoidance of chronic illness and increased lifespan. Given that autophagy activity usually declines with age, fasting may be a natural strategy to boost it. Autophagy is one of the benefits of intermittent fasting, but there are other more intriguing study discoveries, such as the following:

Weight Loss

Large number of research has shown the effectiveness of intermittent fasting for weight reduction in women over 60's. Some study shows that women who follow intermittent fasting routines lose the same amount of weight as those who decrease calories without experiencing feelings of deprivation. In terms of

helping women over 60 lose weight and eliminate extra body fat, intermittent fasting is a beneficial lifestyle decision. According to various research papers, adopting an intermittent fasting diet resulted in an average weight reduction of 15 pounds on average. Another thorough assessment of the studies on intermittent fasting discovered that it might decrease the bodyweight of overweight women by up to 8% in as little as three weeks when done consistently.

Increased Fat Burning in Women over 60's

While reducing carbohydrate consumption, the body begins to use other energy sources as a substitute. After using up all carbohydrate reserves, it might turn to fat for fuel. According to some studies, fasting boosts fat burning by activating the metabolic switch, which allows fat to be used as fuel. Consuming food within a certain time frame causes the body to burn more calories during the rest of its working day. Because the longer without eating, the slower the metabolism gets.

However, by restricting the meal consumption to an 8-hour timeframe, a woman's body will step up to the plate and burn more calories throughout the day and night.

The state of one's mind:

Fasting may help to improve cognitive performance, which is particularly important as women reach their 60s. It may also slow down neurodegeneration, which is the steady deterioration of brain cells over time, but this has only been shown in preclinical studies. Several modifiable factors influence cognitive health and the risk of cognitive decline and Alzheimer's disease. These factors include blood glucose and insulin levels and other metabolic and lipid profiles. Intermittent fasting has been proven to improve several of these factors, which may also positively affect cognition. Recent experiments have also shown that fasting on an intermittent basis may be beneficial to the neurologic health of women in their 60s.

Longevity: Since autophagy may promote cellular health by removing old, damaged cells, it may be able to prevent oxidative damage and promote healthy aging in the long run. Intermittent fasting has been shown to increase the length lifespan in women. Researchers have discovered that intermittent fasting may prolong a rodent's lifetime by 33-88 in women.

Cardiovascular health: Fasting may also help to maintain good cholesterol levels, which may lower the chance of developing heart disease. Heart disease is the leading cause of death globally, killing more women than any other illness. Within two months of starting an intermittent fasting strategy, a study of women over 60 discovered that it decreased blood pressure by 6 percent. Additionally, this same research found that intermittent fasting reduced participants' cholesterol by 25 percent while simultaneously lowering their triglycerides by an incredible 32 percent

Insulin resistance and high blood sugar levels: Another benefit is that fasting may be as effective as a calorie-restricted diet for promoting weight loss, insulin production, and insulin resistance reduction, according to research. By decreasing insulin levels and drastically reducing insulin resistance, intermittent fasting may help women reduce their chance of acquiring diabetes in the first place. In a study of 100 women over 60's, intermittent fasting for only six months lowered insulin levels by 29 percent and insulin resistance by 19 percent, respectively.

Studies conducted on healthy individuals have established the magic of intermittent fasting to reduce insulin levels by 21-31 percent and blood sugar levels by 3-6 percent in women with pre-diabetes in about 8-12 weeks has been established in studies conducted on healthy individuals.

Immunity: Through the process of autophagy, fasting may have a beneficial effect on the creation of healthy white blood cells. Irregular fasting is an excellent immune system regulator because it regulates the quantity of cytokine production that is released into the bloodstream.

The cytokines interleukin-6 and tumor necrosis factor-alpha, two of the most important in the body's inflammatory response, work together. According to research, fasting has been demonstrated to inhibit the release of these inflammatory mediators.

The immune system modulation that intermittent fasting offers may also be beneficial for women who suffer from moderate to severe allergies.

Inflammation: Inflammation is a medical term that refers to the body's inflammation.

Several studies have shown that fasting positively affects inflammation and oxidative stress indicators. Intermittent fasting may be more effective than other diets when it comes to decreasing inflammation and improving disorders that are related to inflammation, such as:

- Alzheimer's disease is a kind of dementia.
- Arthritis
- Asthma
- Multiple sclerosis is a disease that affects the nervous system.
- Stroke

Maintain lean muscular tone: Fasting has been shown to assist in maintaining lean muscular tone. Compared to calorie-restricted diets, studies have demonstrated that intermittent fasting is more successful in retaining lean muscle mass than other diets for women over 60's.

Having a healthy amount of lean muscle tone makes the body more fit and appealing and allows it to burn much more calories - even when the body is fully at rest. This is a major benefit of fasting which can help a lot of women over 60 gain confidence.

Psychological and emotional well-being: Another benefit of intermittent fasting is one's psychological and emotional well-being. According to the findings of recent research, merely 8 weeks of intermittent fasting may significantly reduce depression and binge eating behaviors in women in their 60s while simultaneously improving levels of self-esteem. Many women feel happier after fasting, resulting into a better life.

2.2 The Truth about Intermittent Fasting

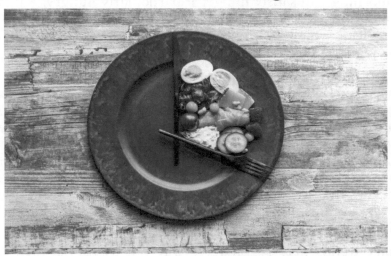

Intermittent fasting is a fantastic strategy to lose weight, and to a certain degree, it may also help enhance metabolic activity. However, according to the data of many researchers, it is not a more effective or faster method of reducing weight when compared to daily calorie restriction but definitely a healthier one. It is necessary to make lifestyle modifications to practice intermittent fasting, and time-restricted fasting is the most practicable strategy for working professionals.

Additionally, intermittent fasting has several health advantages, which may be enhanced even further if being mindful of the food intake throughout the non-fasting time.

Eat high-calorie junk food during the non-fasting window, and the benefits of intermittent fasting may be diminished due to the additional calories consumed. Maintaining a 16-hour fast and consuming high-calorie items such as fries, chips, cakes, and other baked goods may undermine all of the work to maintain a fast. To want to transition to intermittent fasting, make sure to have a well-balanced and healthy meal during the periods when you are not fasting.

For the first few days, it may be difficult to stick to an intermittent fasting schedule since the body is not used to being hungry for such a long time. But if being persistive towards it, the body will develop the habit of missing breakfast for a few of days. Sipping on a cup of black coffee or green tea in the morning will satisfy hunger if particularly hungry. Although these beverages do not promote the production of much insulin, these drinks may help prolong the fasting state while also reducing hunger symptoms.

The truth is that intermittent fasting is not really a solution, but it may benefit certain people who want to achieve their health objectives while maintaining their eating habits. It may thus be an advantageous lifestyle if one does not have any concerns with cravings, migraines, or low sugar levels while on this diet plan. For a woman experiencing any of these symptoms, it is apparent that this is not a healthy solution. Several different approaches to achieving the health objectives do not need adhering to a diet, but it's an intriguing and promising idea to try intermittent fasting.

Dietary trends may be on their way out as people turn their attention to nutrition rather than calories counted to lose weight. Alternatively, it might represent a significant lifestyle constraint, especially if the body of data is still being debated, and it may also have its own set of potentially harmful side effects. As an emerging idea, intermittent fasting requires a longer period of observation and more human trials before it can be recommended.

Please be advised that fasting is not suggested for some groups of individuals, those with a history of eating problems and people with type 1 diabetes. Those considering trying the intermittent fasting diet should speak with their primary care physician and, if possible, with a qualified dietitian before proceedings

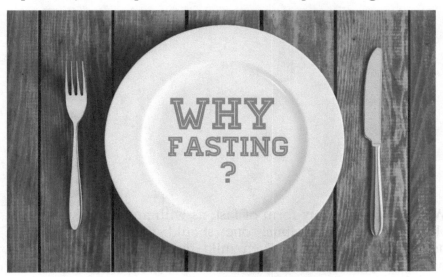

2.3 Why start Intermittent Fasting After the '60s

Many women start practicing intermittent fasting for a variety of different purposes. It might be for several reasons, including weight reduction, improved sleep at night, or increased vitality. One of the most compelling reasons for women over 60 to pursue intermittent fasting is the desire for improved energy. Many women endure a small weight increase and a decrease in the quality of their sleep in their 60s. Both have the potential to make the body feel tired and unproductive. However, by altering the timing and composition of meals, women can retrain the body to function more efficiently.

While fasting to lose weight, intermittent fasting may enable consuming the things that a woman desires when craving them the most — in the middle of the night. In other words, feeling starved when everyone else is nibbling in front of the television while watching their favorite shows will be over.

2.4 How is Intermittent Fasting Riskier for Women over 60?

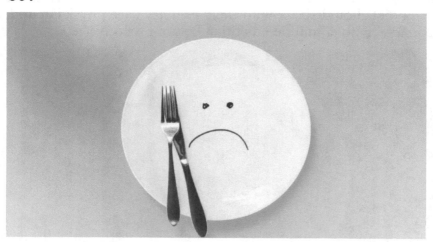

While beginning any form of fast, as with any other substantial change in eating habits, one should first consult with a healthcare practitioner. Even mild fasting may be dangerous, particularly for women who have a history of eating disorders or disordered eating patterns.

- Having diabetes or hypoglycemia may be dangerous, particularly if using drugs that reduce blood sugar.

- Women who are having difficulty gaining enough weight or who are dealing with vitamin deficits.

- A history of electrolyte abnormalities, particularly after fasting for extended periods.

It's not that some women cannot fast if they fall into any of these categories, but it is much more crucial to seek professional counsel to determine whether or not it is safe for them to do so. No words can express how important it is to consult with a trained health practitioner before commencing if diagnosed with a history of disordered eating or an eating disorder. It is possible that the anticipated danger will not occur.

Stress has a significant influence on women's hormones, which accounts for a large portion of the reasons why fasting might be different for them. Intermittent fasting is generally considered to be safe for the majority of individuals. However, investigations have shown that intermittent fasting has certain mild bad impacts. Furthermore, it is not the best option for everyone. The following are the risks of Intermittent Fasting for women in their 60s.

Migraines and dizziness

Intermittent fasting is associated with several unpleasant side effects, including headaches. They are most often experienced during the first several days of a diet program. A study published in 2022 looked at numerous studies, including women over 60 who were on intermittent fasting regimens. Some individuals in the four trials that recorded negative impacts felt slight headaches.

Contrary to popular belief, however, studies have discovered that "fasting headaches" are frequently situated in the brain's frontal area, with the severity of the pain normally being mild to moderate. Furthermore, those who suffer from headaches regularly are more prone than those who do not to suffer from headaches when fasting. Researchers have hypothesized that low caffeine withdrawal and low blood sugar may play a role in headaches in women over 60 s when intermittent fasting.

Exhaustion and a lack of energy

According to studies, some women who follow different techniques of intermittent fasting report exhaustion and a lack of energy on certain occasions. If you suffer from severe adrenal exhaustion, intermittent fasting may make you feel weak. Because your body doesn't have enough adrenaline to control your blood sugar, intermittent fasting might produce low blood sugar (hypoglycemia).

Feeling fatigued and weak due to low blood sugar caused by intermittent fasting is common in women. In addition, intermittent fasting may induce sleep difficulties in certain women, resulting in fatigue throughout the day for those who follow it.

However, several studies have shown that intermittent fasting might actually help to lessen tiredness, particularly when the body gets used to regular fasting intervals.

Hunger pangs

It may come as no surprise that hunger is one of the most prominent negative outcomes associated with intermittent fasting for women over 60's, as it is with any other kind of diet. Women may feel an increased appetite when restricting their calorie intake or going for long durations without consuming calories. Some women in a research were allocated to an intermittent energy restriction group. They ate 440 or 650 calories on two nonconsecutive days per week for a year, depending on their weight.

Participants in these groups reported greater hunger levels than those who followed a low-calorie diet that included continual calorie restriction. Scientists believe that hunger is a symptom that individuals feel during the first few days of starting a fasting program. Another research from 2020 looked at 15 women over 60's who took part in fasting programs that lasted between 4 and 21 days. When they started the regimens, they tended to have severe hunger sensations during the first several days. As a result, sensations such as hunger may subside as the body gets used to frequent fasting intervals.

Inability to control one's temper and other mood swings

Women over 60 who practice intermittent fasting may develop irritation and other mood problems due to their efforts. When the blood sugar is low, women may get irritable. It is possible to have low blood sugar, or hypoglycemia, during times of calorie restriction or during periods of fasting. This might result in irritation, anxiety, and difficulty concentrating on tasks. Research published in 2020 on 52 women over 60 discovered that participants were substantially more irritable after an 18-hour fasting phase than they were during a no fasting time. Interestingly, the researchers discovered that, although the women were more irritable after the fasting period, they also reported a greater feeling of accomplishment, pride, and self-control at the end of the fasting period than they did at the beginning of the fasting period.

Bad Breath

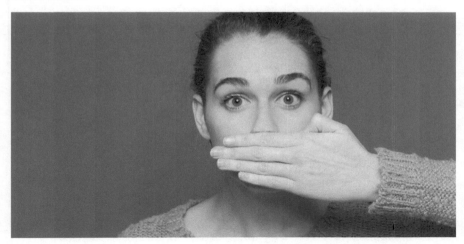

In certain women, bad breath may be a nasty side effect of intermittent fasting, which can be particularly uncomfortable. This is caused by a loss of salivary flow and an increase in the amount of acetone in the breath. Fasting helps your body to burn fat as fuel, which is beneficial. Acetone is a by-product of fat metabolism, and as a result, it accumulates in the blood and exhaled breath while fasting. Dehydration is also a side effect of intermittent fasting and may also produce dry mouth, exacerbating foul breath.

Digestive problems

Symptoms of intermittent fasting include diarrhea, nausea, bloating and constipation. While fasting, the decrease in food consumption associated with certain intermittent fasting regimens may severely impact digestion, resulting in constipation and other adverse effects.

Furthermore, dietary modifications connected with intermittent fasting routines may result in bloating and diarrhea. Constipation might worsen due to dehydration, which is another typical adverse effect of intermittent fasting. As a result, it is critical to maintaining enough hydration when engaging in intermittent fasting.

Constipation may be prevented by eating meals that are high in nutrients and fiber.

Disturbed Sleep

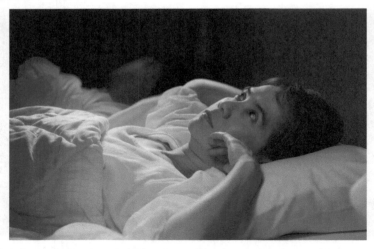

While intermittent fasting tends to increase sleep quality, depending on how meals are timed, it may also cause sleep problems. Women' s sleep might be disrupted when they eat at odd hours. This is particularly true if individuals eat late at night, since this may cause the body's temperature to rise, which is the polar opposite of what happens when sleeping. Heavy meals eaten too soon at night may upset the stomach and make it difficult to fall asleep, resulting in poor sleep quality and a lack of energy when one wakes up.

Moreover, Sleep disruptions, such as the inability to fall asleep or remain asleep, are among the most prevalent negative effects associated with intermittent fasting, such as insomnia for women over 60. As the body excretes huge quantities of salt and water via the urine during the first few days of an intermittent fasting diet, fatigue may be more typical during those first few days.

Dehydration and low sodium levels might occur as a result. Other research, on the other hand, has shown that intermittent fasting has no impact on sleep in women over 60's.

Dehydration

During the first few days of fasting, the body excretes enormous volumes of water and salt via the urine, which is a sign of dehydration. Natural diuresis, also known as natriuretic of fasting, is the term used to describe this process. If this occurs and does not replenish the fluids and electrolytes lost through urine, the person may become dehydrated. In addition, women who practice intermittent fasting may forget to drink or may not drink enough water during their fasting periods. This is particularly likely to occur at the start of an intermittent fasting routine.

To get through a lengthy fast, many individuals depend on caffeine in coffee (or flavored coffee). While this isn't always a problem, the fact remains that coffee is a diuretic. In other words, it has the potential to cause dehydration. That's why drink plenty of water throughout the day and keep an eye on the urine color to ensure that the body is well hydrated. A light lemonade hue is an ideal choice for this. If your urine is dark in color, it may indicate that you are dehydrated.

Poor Nutrition

Intermittent fasting, if not done appropriately, may result in nutritional deficiency. It is possible to become malnourished if a woman fasts for an extended length of time and do not refill their body with sufficient nutrients. Women who participate in different forms of intermittent fasting programs can often satisfy their calorie and nutritional requirements. However, if someone doesn't properly plan and implement the fasting program over a long time, or if they purposely limit calories to an excessive degree, they may suffer from malnutrition and other health problems.

It is important to have a well-balanced, healthy diet when engaging in intermittent fasting. Make certain not to restrict calorie intake excessively. A healthcare practitioner with extensive knowledge in intermittent fasting can assist at the start of intermittent fasting in developing a safe strategy that offers a suitable number of calories and the proper quantities of nutrients for your specific nutritional needs.

However, many of these symptoms can be reduced by making modest modifications, such as reducing the length of time to fast. Having said that, some individuals just do not feel good when fasting, and which is perfectly acceptable.

The disadvantages outweigh the advantages

If you've come this far and decide to fast, it's a good idea to think about how you can do it securely. Here are some steps you can take to get started.

Begin with little steps. If you've never fasted before, you shouldn't go into an extensive fast without some preparation. Begin by simply extending the time between supper and breakfast by a few minutes more than customary. Even ten hours is wonderful if you're used to grazing throughout the evening. Because digestion and insulin function generally slow down as the day progresses, it may be good to start eating supper one hour earlier than you are used to each evening.

Make sure you drink plenty of water. While fasting may imply that you don't consume any calories, calorie-free fluids such as water and herbal tea are advised. Drinking plenty of water can alleviate headaches and hunger pangs in some people. Furthermore, since we satisfy a portion of our overall fluid requirements via water-containing meals, you may need to drink more to make up for lost fluids depending on how long your fast lasts.

Make a plan ahead of time. Make sure you have delicious, healthful things ready to eat when you decide to break your fast. Choose a lunch that is high in healthy fats, protein, and complex carbohydrates for optimum blood sugar balance, and use that meal to set the tone for the remainder of the day. As a source of inspiration, you may consult our free hormone balancing recipe guide.

Keep physical activity to a bare minimum. The length of your fast may dictate how much of an increase in intensity you should do throughout your workout session. Shorter fasts may not necessarily impair your capacity to exercise, but lengthier fasts may need the use of walking or easy yoga as a substitute for vigorous activity.

Pay attention to your body. You're not feeling well when you're fasting? Don't try to push it. If you aren't feeling well, there is simply no need for you to continue your fasting regimen. You are the most knowledgeable about your own body. Don't try to push it; repeat after me.

Chapter 3: Types Of Intermittent Fasting

There are numerous intermittent fasting strategies, ranging in the fasting period: from a twelve-hour overnight fast to a whole-day fast. Methods with a shorter fasting time are well-suited for newbies. Longer fasting times give additional rewards and are suggested for experienced fasters. The first step is to figure out how to make intermittent fasting work for oneself, especially when it comes to things like going out with friends or exercising, so that you don't miss out on important things. Following are different types of intermittent fasting that you can follow.

3.1 A weekly 24-hour Fast

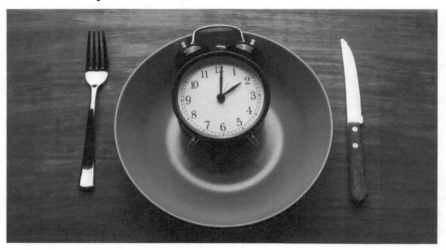

This intermittent fasting pattern, also known as the Eat-Stop-Eat diet, entails going without meals for periods of up to 24 hours at a time. Many individuals fast from one meal to the next, such as from breakfast to breakfast or lunch to lunch.

On days when one is not fasting, one may eat according to a normal schedule. A person's overall calorie intake is reduced due to eating in this way, but the particular items that the individual eats are not restricted.

A 24-hour fast may be very difficult because of the weariness, headaches, and irritation that may accompany it. But people get used to this new dietary pattern over time, and they begin to enjoy the advantages as a result. Weekly 24-hour fasting is one of the most popular methods of adopting intermittent fasting into one's lifestyle. It entails limiting food and drink consumption for a whole day (24 hours) once every week but still consuming all of the nutrients the body requires on all the other days of the week.

When one fasts for 24 hours, they can reflect on themselves and practice self-discipline without experiencing any negative consequences of long periods of fasting, such as hunger or dehydration, that can occur with long periods of absence from food and liquid consumption. It is significant to mention that those who are fasting for 24 hours may continue to consume water, tea, and other calorie-free beverages throughout their fasting time. It is a crucial component of this diet plan. This may seem to be a difficult task.

However, breaking it down into smaller steps is pretty manageable. In the evening before the fasting day, one can eat supper and retire for the night. As soon as the supper is complete, the 24-hour fast period will officially start. The fast for the week is fulfilled the next day when one skips breakfast and lunch and then has a wonderful nutritious supper to round off the day. After a non-fasting day, one must return to their usual eating habits and resume their normal meal times. Eating in this manner decreases a person's overall calorie consumption without restricting the kind of meals that the individual eats.

Pros: The benefits of a 24-hour fast include the fact that it is straightforward to follow and its effectiveness in aiding with weight reduction. It puts courage and mental fortitude to the test.

Cons: A 24-hour fast may be draining and exhausting, and it can also produce weariness and headaches. Some individuals discover that their body's response to their new dietary patterns becomes less dramatic over time as they grow used to their new eating habits.

Beginning with little steps is the greatest way to succeed: attempt skipping one meal every day until having the motivation to spending a complete day without consuming anything at all. This following kind might be appropriate if one desire's to live a better lifestyle but isn't sure where to begin with.

3.2 12 hours a day Fast

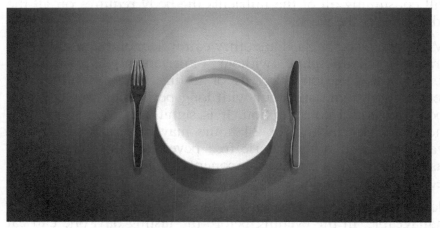

In this type followers typically fast for half of the day and then feast for the remaining 12-hour period of the day. In addition, the hours are flexible. From 8.30 am to 8:30 p.m., 10 am to 10:00 pm, and so on, one may eat at any time. The individual must decide to keep the period that has fast. This category of intermittent fasting is ideal for those who are just getting started. The fasting gap is somewhat shorter than usual. The majority of fasting takes place after the night has gone. It is possible to devour it all at the same moment. For example, one might fast between 6:00 p.m. and 6:00 a.m. or between 6:00 pm and 6:00 a.m. They would have to eat their meal by 6 p.m. and then wait for the next day to start.

Also, considering that one sleeps 7 to 9 hours out of those twelve hours, this type is pretty straightforward to complete. The person who is fasting will likely be sleeping at a time when she may relax. The quickest and most convenient approach to complete the fast is to sleep throughout the timeframe. Finally, the 12-Hour Fast is advised as an excellent starting point for those who are new to intermittent fasting.

Pros: Since it has a smaller period, this style of fasting is simpler to adhere to than others. It may also be beneficial for people who are currently experiencing difficulty sleeping at night and looking for a different solution to enhance their sleep quality.

Cons: Because the fasting period is shorter (just 12 hours), some individuals may not see the same weight-loss advantages as others who engage in lengthier fasting regimens. This kind of intermittent fasting may also cause weariness, particularly if you are exercising when you are not permitted to eat anything.

3.3 Fasting for 16 hours

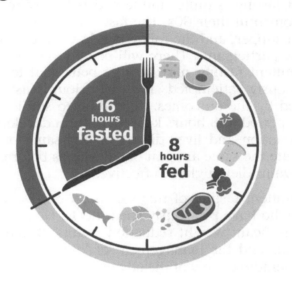

Known as the "birthplace of intermittent fasting," Martin Berkhan developed Leangains in the year 2000. As well as "the Khan, godfather, or high priest of intermittent fasting," Martin is also known as "the Khan." Leangains recommends that one should consume all of the daily calories in 8 hours and fast for the remaining 16 hours of the day. It is the case designed primarily for fitness and strength training and those wishing to achieve the best potential body composition and strength. Compared to other intermittent fasting-based diets, a greater focus is placed on good nutrition before and after workouts.

This involves eating higher-protein foods and consuming more calories on training days while consuming fewer calories on rest days, among other things. The 16:8 fasting method is one of the most popular kinds of intermittent fasting since it is simple to implement into one's everyday routine. In this diet one confines their eating to an eight-hour window with two to three meals and then fast for 16 hours. Example: Eat until 7 pm after supper, then delay breakfast until 11 am the next day, then eat for 8 hours, and the process begins all over again. In this diet we may adjust the time that suits our needs. One may want to eat sooner or later in the day, depending on the schedule.

This sort of fasting is quite simple and is highly recommended for most women in their 60s. The fast is normally completed by 7 p.m. with supper, and the following day, there is no breakfast eaten by the participants. There will be no food served till noon. This intermittent fasting may also be beneficial for those who have previously attempted the 12 Hour Fast and were disappointed by the outcomes. According to studies, restricting the feeding period to 8 hours kept them from developing obesity and inflammation and liver disease in the same proportion as when they ate the same amount of calories as before. Diets such as the Leangains diet might be effective.

Pros: Intermittent fasting of this sort is an excellent alternative for people who have previously tried the 12 Hour Fast but have not seen significant weight reduction results. It may also aid in muscle repair and the management of low blood glucose after exercises, including a few of the advantages.

Cons: This kind of fast is not recommended since it only lasts for a maximum of 16 hours first before women can eat again. Some individuals may be able to stick to this diet more successfully than others because they do not eat numerous meals throughout the day, which causes them to feel unproductive or exhausted.

3.4 The Warrior Diet

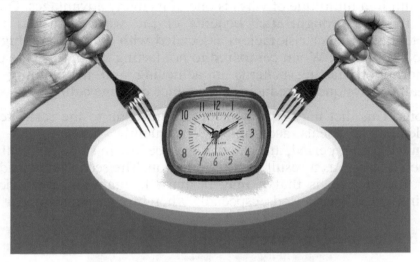

This diet is a twenty-hour fasting phase during which one consumes just a few portion sizes per day before having a huge meal before going to bed. This is a fairly intensive kind of fasting since one is not permitted to consume food or any meals during the day until supper. The body will fast for twenty hours every day in order to practice the warrior diet, excluding one four-hour eating period where one will eat only healthy foods. This kind of fasting may help with mental clarity, weight loss, stress reduction, and the formation of muscle mass.

On the other side, this plan may be too tough for some people to stick to since it requires just a few meals per day and little food on such days. According to its founder, Ori Hofmekler, The Warrior Diet may not be ideal for beginners. The warriors fast for over twenty hours a day and eat just one heavy meal at night. On the other side, fasting allows only a small number of whole foods, fruits, meats, and vegetables.

This diet has been based on common ideas with the Paleo diet. Instead of processed items, it encourages individuals to eat real meals, including meat, chicken, fish, vegetables, and whole grains.

Pros: The fact that a warrior diet is advantageous to overall health in a multitude of ways is one of its many advantages. One of the most sought-after benefits of the warrior diet is its potential to lower risk factors associated with diabetes and high blood pressure. When compared to not fasting at all, this type of intermittent fasting benefits in achieving and maintaining a healthy physique by reducing the chance of binge eating.

Cons: This diet may be tough to continue due to the restricted selection of meals accessible. Consequently, women have a limited eating period, and the diet may be low in some nutrients, such as fiber, as a result of this limitation. The second downside of this lifestyle is that it may be hard to maintain a warrior mindset for long periods, especially when hunger pains appear.

3.5 Alternate Day Fasting

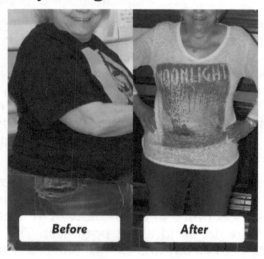

Alternate day fasting is a kind of intermittent fasting taken to the extreme. As the name implies, fasting every other day is part of this regimen. Food is confined to a single 500-calorie meal or complete fasting on fasting days, depending on the situation (without calories). On alternate days, one may eat as they usually would. Alternate day fasting is a difficult type of fasting that is unlikely to be sustained in the long run. Alternate day fasting is a practice in which individuals abstain from eating solid meals on alternate days.

It is important to note that alternate-day fasting is a very severe type of intermittent fasting, and it may not be appropriate for women who have never fasted before or for those who have certain medical concerns. Beginners experiencing medical troubles may wish to avoid using this fasting technique. Additionally, it may be difficult to maintain a consistent fasting approach for an extended period.

Some studies, however, have indicated that alternate-day fasting may result in significant weight reduction, improved digestive and immunological health, and improved metabolic health. One research estimated that 32 individuals dropped an average of about 10 pounds over 12 weeks. Over the study's 12 weeks, 32 individuals dropped a total of 5.3 kg. According to reliable sources, it was also proven to be beneficial for reducing weight and improving heart health in healthy and overweight women.

For some individuals, an alternative diet is consuming foods that are not solid.

Pros: This diet may be useful for weight reduction and improving health indicators such as blood pressure and cholesterol levels.

Cons: Even if one is a rookie or has medical concerns that would make this harmful, it is incredibly tough to go through this form of fasting. It may also take up to 12 weeks before one see any noticeable improvements.

3.6 5:2 Method

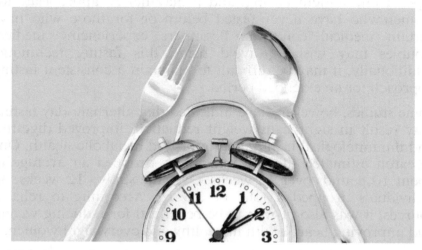

Michael Mosley is recognized for popularizing the 5:2 intermittent fasting method, often referred to as The Fast Diet. This strategy involves restricting calorie intake to 25% of daily needs on 2 days each week while eating properly on the remaining days. Five days of the week are defined as "normal dining days," as the term indicates. The last two days have calorie limits of 450 to 560 per day. Most people split the two fasting days to avoid the hungry specific symptoms with a two-day fast. During the 2 days of fasting, women intake approximately 400 calories each day.

Women usually adhere to this diet by spacing out regular fasting days all week. As a result, individuals may fast on Tuesdays and Friday while eating normally the rest of the week. To ensure proper digestion, at least one free day should be included between fasting days. This diet, sometimes called also as Fast Diet, has gotten very little research attention. The study included 110 women over the age of 60 and found that caloric intake restriction once a week and constant calorie counting both resulted in similar weight loss.

Among the most apparent benefits was that blood sugar levels decreased considerably, allowing patients to lose weight and improve.

Pros: This meal plan is easily understandable and has been demonstrated to help people lose weight while also lowering their insulin levels.

Cons: Sticking to this kind of fasting may be more challenging since it may experience hunger and be unable to find food throughout the fast.

3.7 Meal Skipping

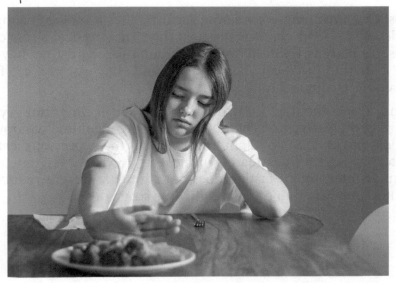

This diet is ideal for individuals who do not want to feel confined or who get disappointed if they do not satisfy the requirements of a certain diet plan.

In it just allow oneself to miss meals if not hungry or too busy to prepare a meal. Cooking and eating take up a great amount of time, and adopting this method of eating can free up the time to devote to other activities—for example, one might substitute a meal with something they like doing, such as going on a walk or practicing yoga. A common misconception is that we must eat three meals a day, and spontaneous meal cutting is an excellent approach to deconstruct this assumption. One will not go hungry if they miss a meal now and then! This intermittent fasting technique is adaptable, which may be beneficial for beginners.

To maintain a certain degree of hunger or to meet time constraints, the individual decides which meals to forego. Individuals who exercise self-control over their appetites are more likely to be effective at meal switching. When one opts to skip meals, it is important to remember to consume nutritious items while doing so, such as fresh vegetables, to keep the energy levels up. The simplest approach to describe meal skipping is to say that to eat when hungry and skip meals when are not hungry, as explained above.

Pros: One advantage of missing meals is that it makes it simpler to develop a food plan for the next day. The physical stress on a person's body is reduced since they don't feel as if they have to "do" anything to eat healthfully, and the variety of food selections is almost limitless.

Cons: Cons include individuals reporting feeling hungry or limiting themselves to specific meals during mealtime windows - which might lead to them reverting to their previous eating patterns and routines (eating unhealthy foods). Over time, this form of intermittent fasting does not stimulate weight reduction in the same way that other weight-loss strategies do.

Chapter 4: How to Start Intermittent Fasting?

4.1 Set Your Smart Goals

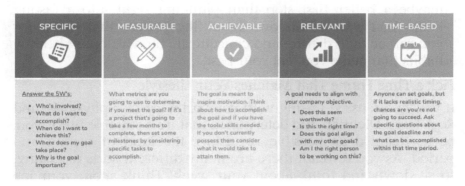

When beginning a new healthy habit, it's vital to consider what obstacles one could encounter. This is an important stage in creating SMART goals, which health coaches use to help clients create realistic, long-term objectives. People have a few frequent issues or questions when it comes to intermittent fasting:

- When I'm not fasting, what do I eat?
- What should I do if I'm feeling queasy or dizzy?
- Is it safe to fast for short periods?
- Should I do an intermittent fast for a certain amount of time?

Understand why you're doing it and assess your current diet

Consider what you want to achieve by incorporating intermittent fasting into your lifestyle:

- Improved dietary habits
- keep track of your blood sugar
- Loss of body weight

- Establish deliberate eating habits, such as eating more thoughtfully.

Whatever your motivation for beginning, examine your present diet and ask yourself what about it is keeping you from achieving the objective you envisioned before. Simple modifications, such as eating a healthy breakfast or learning to calculate macros to better understand portion management, maybe a better first step than plunging right into a fasting habit. You want to discover an eating pattern that works for you rather than dieting and concentrate on developing healthy habits that make you feel your best.

Pick a Time Frame That Matches Your Lifestyle

If you've discussed fasting with your primary care physician and Registered Dietitian and determined that it's a suitable fit for you, be as detailed as possible regarding the kind of fasting and period. As you've read, there are many different sorts of fasting, so sit down and think about your week. Think about your job schedule, sleep pattern, and lifestyle when deciding on a fasting plan.

Begin Small

Start modestly if you're new to occasionally fasting. Choose one day every week to experiment with the style you think would work best for you. For many individuals, short-term fasting is a more sustainable option. Start with an overnight fast of 8-12 hours, which is easy to fit into your schedule, then work your way up to lengthier fasting days. If you're going to fast for a long time, choose a day of the week or a period when you won't need to be especially active or concentrated.

Maintain Hydration

Even if you're fasting, you should drink enough no caloric fluids, particularly water, to keep hydrated. Sugar-free herbal teas and sparkly waters may also be included. Half your body weight in ounces is the recommended quantity of water to drink every day.

If you weigh 160 pounds, you should drink at least 80 ounces of water every day.

Establish a Meal Preparation Routine

Intermittent fasting, if not done effectively, may lead to weight gain. When you're fasting, you may feel starving, making you more prone to binge eating when you're not fasting. Even if you fast for 12-16 hours each day, consuming more calories than your body burns will result in a long-term gain in body fat. To put it another way, if you have difficulties controlling your appetite and go fully wild during your non-fasting times, you may gain weight. Plan your meals ahead of time to ensure you have nutrient-dense options throughout your non-fasting hours and keep below your daily calorie restriction.

You should think about what sort of meal plan you love throughout your non-fasting times since intermittent fasting does not substitute good eating. Do you want more plant-based, vegetarian, vegan, or vegetarian meals? Do you want to go keto? Or do you like to strike a balance with a flexitarian diet? Whatever you choose, have a plan for what you'll eat throughout the non-fasting time.

Make a point of eating well-balanced meals.

When intermittent fasting, the quality of your meal is critical and controlling your blood sugar might be the key to success. Plan your meals ahead of time to ensure you eat nutrient-dense foods throughout your non-fasting hours. Ensure you're getting all of the nutrients you need to keep your body going while you're fasting!

Consuming meals that are balanced with nutritious whole foods, proteins, and fats regularly throughout your non-fasting phase to keep you full and content while avoiding processed sweets and carbs. You may also attempt intuitive eating, which shifts your attention away from calories and willpower and toward understanding what your body needs to flourish, independent of the time of day or when your next allowed eating window is.

To set yourself up for success, remember to integrate fundamental nutrition concepts such as calorie management and a balanced diet, whatever your reason for choosing the intermittent fast.

4.2 Deal with Hunger Pangs

It is no surprise that hunger is constant throughout intermittent fasting, and you may expect it to be far worse during regular fasting. This, however, is not always the case in practice. Hunger lasts around 20 minutes, although most people are unaware of this since they do not wait to discover it. This book will provide you with practical suggestions for preventing hunger pains when fasting.

Some individuals never experience true hunger since their appetite keeps them eating and staying satisfied constantly. True hunger is characterized by stomach grumbling and discomfort caused by the physical urge to consume food. While fasting, it is totally natural to experience hunger. The most difficult aspect is coming up with ideas for your next dinner. Hunger is a conditioned stimulus-response reaction that an individual may recondition.

What is the root cause of hunger?

Appetite is defined as the urge to consume food that is driven by hormones, senses, or feelings. When you are hungry, your hunger sends messages to your brain, but not all of these signals are beneficial to you. When you see something that looks delicious, your body may be led to hunger even after you've finished your meal.

So, what is the source of hunger?

Ghrelin, the hunger hormone, is responsible for the sensation of hunger. When your body is expecting a meal, it releases the hormone ghrelin. Ghrelin is mostly released by the stomach, although it is also released in minor amounts by the pancreas and small intestine. When the hormone is discharged into the circulation, it affects the hypothalamus, which is positioned below the eyes and under the midline of the cerebral cortex. A person will feel the desire to eat as a result of this. Food consumption may be increased by up to 30% due to the hormone cortisol.

The first few days of your fast will be difficult since the want to eat will be continuous throughout the day.

While fasting, you may experience hunger pains. Following are some ways to cope with these sensations while fasting.

How to Fight Hunger While Fasting: 8 Simple Steps?

Because the body is used to regular meals, the system does not expect the change when you begin intermittent fasting. The urge to eat is associated with the reward system of the brain. Hunger may manifest itself not just on a physical level but also on a cognitive one.

Keeping your appetite under control will allow you to maintain your fasting routine. Fortunately, there are a variety of strategies you may use to combat hunger when you are fasting.

Keep Yourself Hydrated.

The body has a tendency to confuse the sensation of thirst with that of hunger. When you're hungry, you may be merely thirsty. Drinking water immediately after waking up will allow you to get a jump start on your hydration intake. Consume two to three liters of water every day, if at all possible. Staying hydrated helps you feel fuller for longer periods of time. However, excessive water consumption may cause valuable electrolytes to be flushed from the body, resulting in dehydration. Drinking lots of water is one of the most important tools you can use to keep your fast going.

Approximately 30% of the water you consume comes from your diet. Therefore, you should account for this while fasting intermittently. To prevent eating and keep within your fasting objectives, you might add appetite suppressants to your water. If you find it difficult to drink plain sparkling water, you may add fasting vitamins to your drink to make it more bearable. Carbonated water is another one of the hacks that may be used when on a fast. In addition to having zero calories, it also includes carbon dioxide, which causes you to feel full when it fills your stomach. You may also take apple cider vinegar as a supplement while you're on an intermittent fasting schedule. Apple cider vinegar (ACV) provides several health advantages while also keeping your content without requiring you to break your fast.

Taking apple cider vinegar in the morning or just before having a meal helps to absorb minerals from the meals you ate before the fast began. If you don't like the flavor of apple cider vinegar, try ACV gummies.

Get A Good Night's Sleep

Your appetite will be affected if you have irregular sleeping habits, are stressed, or use alcohol. It is important to go to bed and wake up early. Your blood sugar levels and hormones are also affected by poor sleep habits. These actions will cause hormone-induced hunger, prompting you to break your fast. You can control your hormone levels by getting adequate sleep, drinking less alcohol, and using stress-reduction tactics. For improved sleep quality, you need a comfortable and well-ventilated bedroom.

It's also crucial to go to bed early and keep to a regular sleeping schedule in a peaceful setting. You should also avoid watching television before going to bed. You should minimize your alcohol intake as much as possible before beginning your fasting phase. This stabilizes your blood sugar levels and reduces unpredictable hormones.

Fasting Hours Should Be Scheduled Overnight

A 10–16-hour fast has been shown to induce the body to begin burning fat into energy from its stores, according to research. By releasing ketones into the body, promotes weight loss. It is a great way to get started with intermittent fasting. The fasting window is short, and one may eat the same number of calories every day.

The ideal strategy to complete a 10–16-hour fast is to do it during your nocturnal sleeping hours. For example, your eating schedule may be from 7 a.m. until 7 p.m.

A mouse research found that time-restricted feeding protected mice against metabolic illnesses like diabetes and obesity, even when they ate the same number of calories as mice that ate anytime they wanted.

Consume Warm Liquids

Warm drinks, such as tea and coffee, assist your body to adjust to the fasting experience rapidly. According to research published by the National Center for Biotechnology Information, catechins (antioxidants found in tea) lower ghrelin release. A hot beverage fills the gaps left by eating by making you feel satisfied. Black coffee is healthy as long as it is served without milk or sugar. You should also avoid milk and sugar when drinking tea since they contain calories.

You should be aware that some herbal teas include fruit sweeteners. It would be beneficial if you drank just zero-calorie green tea. If you're having trouble sticking to your intermittent fasting plan, consider bulletproof coffee, which is black coffee mixed with fats such as ghee, butter, or coconut oil. Healthy fats may aid in keeping you in ketosis. If you're a fasting purist, then, you should completely avoid calories since even one more calorie will force you to break your fast.

Do a Little Exercising

When fasting, any kind of physical exercise is beneficial as long as it is done in moderation. Short bursts of activity can divert your attention away from eating.

Walking, yoga, or pilates are all fantastic ways to burn fat, build muscle, and tone down hunger sensations. When you play tennis, basketball, or football, it fools your mind into thinking you're not fasting. The brain concentrates on both exercise and activities.

Walking works practically every muscle group in your body, increasing fat-burning potential. Walking helps your general health while also urging your body to burn fat for energy.

Distract Yourself

When we keep occupied on specific situations, it helps us cope with growing hunger levels. When our bodies anticipate a meal, we may feel hungry at meal times. You may keep yourself engaged by planning workouts or other things to keep you busy. Allowing boredom to sneak in will almost certainly lead to hunger.

Because emotional hunger is linked to physical hunger, boredom leads to overeating. You may make an intermittent fasting strategy and schedule your time accordingly. You may start your day with some housework instead of breakfast. You may also schedule your work meetings around when you eat your lunch. Chewing gum is another strategy to distract yourself from hunger symptoms, but it should only be used as a last option. Sugar-free gum is the greatest alternative since it will not break your fast. Chewing gum momentarily relieves hunger, but it may cause you to get hungry again in the long term.

As you come closer to your eating window, chewing gum is a good idea since the chewing sensation signals to your stomach that you'll be receiving food soon.

When you're not fasting, eat protein-rich, high-fat foods.

Implementing a protein-rich and higher healthier fat diet is the greatest method to lay the groundwork for a low-carb diet. A high-fat, protein-rich diet can help you achieve your weight-loss objectives quicker. Between fasts, sticking to a protein-rich meal stabilizes blood sugar and makes you feel more satiated.

You'll find that your intermittent fasting goes more easily, and you'll feel less hungry.

When you're not fasting, stay away from carbs.

When you're not fasting, one of the diet modifications you should make is to reduce your carb consumption. Intermittent fasting isn't an excuse to consume low-quality food; rather, it's a strategy to make the most of your health and diet.

Following a low-carbohydrate diet keeps you satisfied and your blood sugar in check. Sugary foods elevate blood glucose levels and induce insulin release, which triggers the secretion of hunger hormones even more. Carbs may be replaced with legumes, nutritious grains, and vegetables, which can keep you satisfied for a long time.

4.3 Practice Portion Control

Top nutritionists, dieters, and those attempting to try intermittent fasting all talk about portion management. Restaurants and other food establishments have distorted our perception of what is a portion of a main meal or snack. Furthermore, few individuals understand the need of portion control while dining out and at home. Many people assume that portion control equates to perpetual hunger, but this is not the case.

Portion management does not mean that you should take just a few bites of everything on your plate. It entails consuming the quantity of food required by your body. Managing your meal amounts can help you discover you consume more than your body requires, whether you're on a fast or just want to start eating better.

Make mindful eating a habit.

When you eat thoughtfully, you won't have that awful tummy sensation after a meal. It also helps you to appreciate the tastes and sensations that each item provides. It's difficult to concentrate only on your meal when there are so many distractions, such as cellphones with social networking platforms, computers with important tasks, and televisions with beloved movies.

Eat slowly and thoroughly, chewing your meal well. You'll eat less and feel fuller without overeating this way. The issue is that it takes a long for your stomach to convey a message to your brain that it's full — generally 15 to 20 minutes.

Get up earlier in the morning to intentionally consume your breakfast, and take your time in the evening to really appreciate your supper. It's also been shown that mindful eating may help with bloating and stomach discomfort.

Switch plates.

The more food on your plate, the bigger it is. Even if you just place a little amount of your food on it, your eye will send a signal to your brain and stomach that it's insufficient. Don't let this happen by replacing the dishes you've been using to serve your meals with smaller ones.

That's the ruse restaurants employ to deceive us into ordering more, eating more, and spending more than we need to. They offer colossal dishes with a little quantity of food on them. You immediately assume it's too little for you and that you need to get more.

If you're eating at home, use tiny plates and pile your food. This is the simplest approach to fool your eyes into thinking you're consuming a large amount of food. When dining out, request that your meal be served on tiny plates as well. It's what famous people do when they go out to eat.

Select treats that require peeling, shelling, or unwrapping.

Pistachios, asparagus, oranges, grapefruit, kiwifruit, carrots, walnut and a variety of other foods that take some effort before eating are wonderful snack options. The length of time you spend peeling or shelling provides your stomach time to transmit a "satisfaction" signal to your brain, which helps you avoid overeating. Don't peel anything while preparing your lunch for work; save it for your lunch break.

Begin with a salad.

This method works in both restaurants and at home. If you want to lose a lot of weight, you should try to cut down on bad fats as much as possible. Starting your meal with a bowl of low-calorie, high-greens salad will quell your appetite and cause you to consume less greasy meals.

The same applies for desserts: before ordering your favorite pie, choose a fruit salad without dressings. Green salads are high in nutrients and antioxidants, which help you lose weight and feel and look better by reducing chronic stress, reducing inflammation, and enhancing vitality.

Avoid eating from a package or bag.

If you carefully study a food label, you'll see information on how many calories and grams are in each serving. Take pretzels for example: 10 twists (about 60 grams) have roughly 230 calories.

Consider how many twists are in each package and how many you consume in one sitting the same may be said for whole-wheat crisps or other diet-friendly treats found at the shop.

Before you start eating, read the labels and calculate the portions and calories. Divide the contents of a box or bag into many pieces. Put them in little containers or zip-top bags and eat one anytime you're hungry.

Use a kitchen scale to measure your food if there is no information regarding portions. It may seem absurd, but it's an easy method to figure out how many grams or ounces make up one serving.

Before a meal, drink a glass of water.

When it comes to losing weight reduction, water is a fantastic weapon. It makes you feel filled faster and helps you avoid cravings. Not to mention that it provides you with extra energy, allowing you to work out more vigorously. A common suggestion is to drink a lot of water before each meal, but many people disregard it because they follow it incorrectly.

The key is to drink plenty of water and wait at least 10 minutes before eating. If you need to drastically reduce your calorie intake, drink water after each three spoons of food. When you're hungry, a glass of water can assist you figure out whether your body is craving food or if you're merely thirsty. Many individuals confuse thirst for hunger and eat when they really only need a glass of water.

Bring your meal to your pals to share.

Restaurants tend to provide enormous quantities; so, why not reduce your calorie intake whilst saving money by sharing your food with family or friends? It's much better if they're also keeping track of their servings.

If you don't have somebody to share your meal with, you might ask a server to bring you half a dish. Mindful eating is the key to portion management. It's all about eating for your health, not your waistline. It may take a long time and a lot of patience to figure out how to eat your proper meal quantity, but don't give up and allow space for errors.

Chapter 5: Breakfast Recipes For Intermittent Fasting

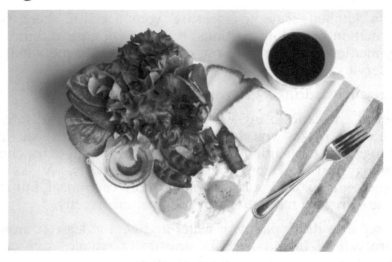

5.1 Fat Burning Green Smoothie

Prep Time: 5 minutes
Cook Time: 5 minutes
Servings: 1
Ingredients

- 1 large ripe banana

- 1 cup roughly chopped mature kale

- 1 big ripe banana

- ¼ ripe avocado

- 1 tablespoon of chia seeds

- 1 cup vanilla unsweetened almond milk

- 2 tablespoons of fresh honey

- 1 pound of ice cubes

Instructions

1.   Combine the kale, banana, chia seeds, almond milk, avocado, and honey in a blender.

2.   Blend on high until smooth and creamy.

3.   Blend in the ice until it is completely smooth.

Nutrition Facts
Fat 14.2g; Protein 5.9g; Sodium 198.9mg.

5.2 Low Carb Pancakes

Prep Time: 30 minutes
Cook Time: 25 minutes
Servings: 6

Ingredients

•   2 teaspoons baking powder

•   ¼ cup sugar-free applesauce

•   1 ½ cups whole-wheat flour

•   2 teaspoons melted coconut oil

•   1 tsp of sugar

•   ¼ teaspoon salt

•   1 ½ cups of unsweetened almond

•   1 tsp vanilla essence

Instructions

1.   Combine flour, baking powder, and salt in a large mixing bowl. Combine the milk, applesauce, oil, sugar, and vanilla in a medium mixing bowl.

2.   Make a well in the middle of the dry ingredients and pour in the wet ingredients, whisking just until combined.

3.   Allow the batter to settle for 10 to 15 minutes without stirring. (The baking powder generates bubbles in the batter while it sits, resulting in fluffy pancakes.)

4.   Cook over medium heat in a large frypan or skillet coated with cooking spray. Using around 1/4 cup batter for each pancake, measure out pancakes and place them onto the pan without mixing the batter (or onto the grill).

5.   Cook for 2 to 4 minutes, or until the edges are dry and bubbles appear on the top. Cook for another 2 to 4 minutes on the other side until golden brown.

6.   Cook the remaining batter in the same way, spraying the pan with cooking spray and lowering the heat as required.

Nutrition Facts
Fat 8.42g; Protein 4.9g; Sodium 10mg

5.3 Keto Tumeric Milkshake

Prep Time: 5 minutes
Cook Time: 5 minutes
Servings: 1
Ingredients

- 1 sugar-free pellet

- 1/2 teaspoon cinnamon 1 sugar-free pellets

- 1 1/2 cup coconut milk

- ice cubes as required

- 1 teaspoon turmeric

- salt as required

- 1/2 teaspoon coconut oil

Instructions

1.   Combine turmeric, ginger, coconut milk, coconut oil, cinnamon, sugar-free pellets, and a bit of salt in a blending jar.

2.   Combine all of the ingredients in a thick milkshake.

3.   Pour into glasses and top with cinnamon powder.

4.   After that, grab a glass and pour the milkshake all the way to the top, then sprinkle some cinnamon and turmeric on top.

5.   You may also throw in a couple of ice cubes just before serving.

Nutrition Facts

Fat; 35g, Protein; 1.6g,

5.4 Breakfast Burritos

Prep Time: 35 minutes
Cook Time: 25 minutes
Servings: 6

Ingredients

- 10 flour tortillas

- 1 (16 ounces) can of refried beans

- 1-pound bacon

- 10 eggs

- 8 ounces shredded Cheddar cheese

Instructions

1.   In a big, deep-pan, cook the bacon.

2.   Cook until uniformly browned over medium-high heat.

3.   Drain the water and put it aside.

4.   Wrap the tortillas in foil and placing them in the oven.

5.   In an oiled skillet, fry the eggs until hard.

6.   Heat the refried beans in a small saucepan.

7.   Refried beans, 2 slices of bacon, 1 egg, and a little cheese go on top of each tortilla.

8.   Serve burritos made with tortillas.

Nutrition Facts

Fat 39.1g; Protein 25.6g Sodium; 1180.9mg.

5.5 Fat-Burning Coconut Cookies

Prep Time: 35 minutes
Cook Time: 25 minutes
Servings: 6

Ingredients

- ¼ cup almond flour

- ¾ cup granular sucralose sweetener

- 3 eggs

- 1 teaspoon almond milk

- ½ cup butter

- ½ tablespoon heavy cream

- 1 teaspoon almond milk

- ½ cup unsweetened coconut flakes

- 6 tablespoons coconut flour

- ¼ cup almond flour

- 1 teaspoon baking powder

Instructions

1.   Preheat the oven to 350°F (180°C) (175 degrees C). Using parchment paper, line a baking sheet.

2.   In a mixing bowl, cream together the sweetener and butter. Combine the eggs, almond milk, and heavy cream in a mixing bowl and whisk until smooth.

3.   With a spatula, scrape down the sides.

4.   Combine baking powder, coconut flakes, baking soda, coconut flour, almond flour, and salt in a separate dish. Mix in the butter until the dough comes together.

5.   Using a teaspoon, drop cookie batter onto baking sheets.

6.   Bake for 17 minutes in a pre-heated oven till golden brown.

7.   Cool for 3 minutes on the baking sheet before transporting it to a wire rack to cool completely.

Nutrition Facts

Fat 8.9g; Protein 2g; Sodium 210.9mg

5.6 Spinach Frittata

Prep Time: 20 minutes
Cook Time: 10 minutes
Servings: 4
Ingredients

- 2 tablespoons extra virgin olive oil

- 1/8 teaspoon freshly ground pepper

- 2 tablespoons chopped sun-dried tomatoes, optional

- 1 large clove of garlic, minced

- 1/4 teaspoon salt

- 2 ounces (56g) of goat cheese

- 1/3 cup (about 1 ounce, 30g) grated Parmesan cheese

- 8 ounces (225g) or more fresh chopped spinach (or use baby spinach)

- 9 large eggs

- 1 medium onion, chopped (about 1 cup)

- 2 tablespoons milk

Instructions

1.   Whisk milk, eggs, & Parmesan cheese in a mixing dish. Add the pepper and salt and mix well. Remove from the equation.

2.   Heat the olive oil over medium heat in an ovenproof, nonstick skillet. Add the onion, then cook for 4 to 5 minutes, or until transparent.

3.   Cook for another minute after adding the garlic and sun-dried tomatoes (if using). A handful of spinach at a time should be added.

4.   Toss in the onion with tongs.

5.   Add additional spinach to the pan when the fresh spinach starts to wilt and create space in the pan. Spread the spinach mixture evenly over the bottom of the pan after it has wilted.

6.   The onion and spinach pour the egg mixture.

7.   Lift the mixture along the pan's sides with a spatula to allow the egg mixture to flow below.

8.   Over the top of the frittata mixture, sprinkle goat cheese chunks.

9.   Reduce to a low heat setting, then cover the pan.

10.   Cook for 10 to 13 minutes on the stovetop, or until everything except the center of the frittata is done. (You may need to check the frittata a few times to see how it's setting.) The wavy center should remain.

11.   Preheat the oven to broil. Place the baking dish in the oven's top third. Broil for 3 minutes, or until golden brown on top.

12.   Remove using oven mitts and set aside to cool for a few minutes.

13.   To serve, cut into wedges.

Nutrition Facts

Fat 21; Protein 23; Sodium 520mg;

5.7 Low-Calorie Porridge

Prep Time: 3 minutes
Cook Time: 7 minutes

Servings: 3
Ingredients

- Berries

- Almond paste

- 50 g oat flakes

- 130 ml water

- 1 pinch of salt

Instructions

1.   Make the water hot in a kettle.

2.   In a bowl, combine the oat flakes and a touch of salt.

3.   Fill the basin halfway with hot water.

4.   Mix the porridge thoroughly until it has a creamy consistency.

5.   Assemble your toppings and place them on top of the porridge.

Nutrition Facts

Fat 0.0g; Protein 2.6; Sodium 52.2mg

Chapter 6: Lunch Recipes For Intermittent Fasting

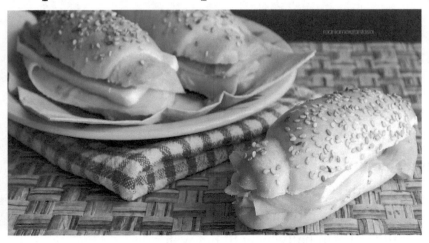

6.1 Jars of Chicken Spring Rolls

Prep Time: 35 minutes
Cook Time: 20 minutes
Servings: 8
Ingredients

- 1-quart oil for deep frying

- 1 small carrot, grated

- ¼ cup barbeque sauce

- 1 dash of soy sauce

- 1 (14 ounces) package spring roll wrappers

- 1 small onion, grated

- 2 (10 ounces) can chunk chicken, drained and flaked

- 1 dash of hot pepper sauce

- 1 dash Worcestershire sauce

- ½ cup finely shredded cabbage

Instructions

1.   Heat the oil to 375 degrees F in a deep-fryer or a big, heavy saucepan (190 degrees C).

2.   Combine the onion, carrot, chicken, hot pepper sauce, barbeque sauce, hot pepper sauce, soy sauce, and Worcestershire sauce in a medium mixing bowl.

3.   1 spoonful of the chicken combination should be placed in the middle of each spring roll wrapper.

4.   Wet your fingers and the edges of the wrapper with water.

5.   Roll the filling around with your hands.

6.   Seams should be pressed together to seal them.

7.   Deep fry the spring rolls in small batches for 4 minutes, or till golden brown.

8.   Using paper towels, absorb any excess liquid.

Nutrition Facts

Fat 13.9g; Protein 16.2g; Sodium 586.8mg

6.2 Zucchini Noodle Casserole

Prep Time: 20 minutes
Cook Time: 40 minutes
Servings: 4

Ingredients

*   5 zucchini squash, cut into the shape of noodles

*   3 tablespoons olive oil

*   salt and black pepper

*   ½ cup shredded mozzarella cheese

*   1 (7 ounces) Greek yogurt

*   18 ounce) jar marinara sauce

*   to taste minced garlic

- 1 pinch of Italian seasoning

- ½ cup shredded mozzarella cheese

Instructions

1. Preheat the oven to 400 degrees Fahrenheit (200 degrees C).

2. In a large skillet, heat 1 oil over medium-high heat. In batches, cook enough zucchini to fill the pan with 1 tablespoon of garlic until softened and slightly browned, 5 to 7 minutes.

3. Using the remaining zucchini, oil and garlic, repeat the process.

4. Fill a baking dish halfway with the cooked zucchini mixture.

5. In a saucepan over low heat, whisk together marinara sauce, yogurt, Italian seasoning, salt, and black pepper; simmer and stir until sauce is warm through, 3 to 5 minutes.

6. In the baking dish, pour the sauce over the zucchini mixture.

7. Over the top, add mozzarella and a touch of Italian spice.

8. Cook for 15 to 25 minutes in a preheated oven until the cheese is melted.

Nutrition Facts
Fat 17.7g; Protein 12g; Sodium 620.1mg.

6.3 Fish Tacos

Prep Time: 20 minutes
Cook Time: 40 minutes
Servings: 4
Ingredients

- cups shredded cabbage

- ½ cup salsa

- 1 teaspoons salt

- 3 lbs. fillets of tilapia

- 1 teaspoon chipotle peppers

- 1 tomato, chopped

- 16 (5 inches) corn tortillas

- 1 tbsp. black pepper

- 1 avocado - sliced

- 1 ½ tbsp fresh cilantro (sliced)

- 2 cups of shredded cheese

- cooking spray

- A teaspoon of paprika

- 2 onions (chopped)

- ½ cup plain fat-free yogurt

- 2 tablespoons lime juice

- 1 tbsp garlic powder

Instructions

1. Season tilapia fillets with salt, garlic powder, black pepper and paprika after rubbing them with 2 tbsp Of lime juice.

2. Using cooking spray, coat both sides of the fillet.

3. Preheat the grill to medium heat and brush the grate gently with oil.

4. In a blender, combine the yogurt, 2 tbsp cilantro, lime juice and chipotle pepper; pulse until thoroughly combined. Set aside.

5. Grill tilapia until it can easily be split using a fork, approximately 6 minutes on a separate side, on a hot grill.

6. In a pan over low heat, cook each corn tortilla for approximately 1 minute. Serve grilled fish with cabbage lime

sauce, cheese, salsa, tomato, avocado, and onions on corn tortillas.

Nutrition Facts

Fat 11g; Protein 31.5g; Sodium 846.7mg

6.4 Lemon Green Beans

Prep time: 5 minutes
Cook time: 25 minutes
Serving: 6

Ingredients

- 1 pound fresh green beans, rinsed and trimmed

- ¼ cup sliced almonds

- 2 teaspoons lemon pepper

- 2 tablespoon butter

Instructions

1.   In a steamer, place green beans over 1 inch of boiling water.

2.   Cook and cover for approximately 10 minutes until it's tender and still firm; drain.

3.   Meanwhile, in a pan over medium heat, melt the butter.

4.   Toast the almonds in a skillet, and season with lemon pepper for taste. Toss in the green beans well enough to coat.

Nutrition Facts

Fat 5.9g; Protein 2.3g; Sodium 185.8mg

6.5 Eggplant Parmesan Panini

Prep time: 25 minutes

Cook time: 45 minutes

Serving: 8

Ingredients

- ½ cup chopped fresh basil

- 8 tablespoons olive oil

- 8 ounces' ricotta cheese

- 1 ½ tablespoons salt

- 4 cups pasta sauce

- 1 eggplant, cut into 3/4 inch slices

- 6 ounces shredded mozzarella cheese

- ½ cup grated Parmesan cheese

- 1 egg, beaten

Instructions

1.   Season the eggplant slices on both sides with salt. Place the slices in a sieve with a dish below to catch the liquid that will evaporate as the eggplant sweats. Allow for 30 minutes of resting time.

2.   Preheat the oven to 350 °F (175 degrees C). Combine the ricotta, mozzarella, and 1/4 cup Parmesan cheese in a medium mixing basin. Combine the egg and basil in a mixing bowl.

3.   Rinse the eggplant well in cold water to eliminate any salt.

4.   4 tablespoons olive oil, heated in a large pan over medium heat brown from each side about one layer of eggplant in the pan. Repeat with the remaining eggplant slices, using more oil as needed.

5.   1 1/2 cups spaghetti sauce, distributed evenly in a 9x13 inch baking dish. On top of the sauce, arrange a layer of eggplant slices. 1/2 of the cheese mixture should be placed on top of the eggplant.

6.   Continue stacking until all of the eggplant and cheese mixtures has been used. Add the remaining sauce over the layers, then top with the leftover Parmesan cheese.

7.   Bake for 30 to 45 minutes, until the sauce, is bubbling, in a preheated oven.

Nutrition Fact

Fat 17.1g; Protein 15g; Sodium 671.6mg

6.6 Paleo Chicken Stew

Prep Time: 15 minutes
Cook Time: 35 minutes
Servings: 6

Ingredients

- 1 cup fresh spinach, or to taste

- 1 small red onion, chopped

- 1 pinch paprika, or more to taste

- sea salt to taste

- 1 pinch crushed red pepper, or more to taste

- 2 teaspoons olive oil

- 2 skinless, boneless chicken breast halves, cut into cubes

- 2 sweet potatoes, peeled and chopped

- ½ cup chicken broth, or more to taste

- 2 cloves garlic, minced

Instructions

1.   In a saucepan, heat the olive oil over medium-high heat. 5 minutes in high oil, sauté onion and garlic until softened.

2.   Combine the sweet potatoes, chicken, spinach, paprika, crushed red pepper, and sea salt with onion and garlic in a saucepan.

3.   Pour chicken stock into the pot to make the mixture soupy or stew.

4.   Bring the stock to a boil, then lower to medium-low heat and cook for 30 minutes, or until the chicken is just no longer pink inside the center and the potatoes are soft.

Nutrition Facts

Fat 2.6g; Protein 9.6g; Sodium 223mg;

6.7 Chicken Salad with Walnuts and Grapes

Prep Time: 25 minutes
Cook Time: 25 minutes
Servings: 4
Ingredients

- 1 ½ tablespoon and ½ teaspoon mayonnaise

- ⅔ Granny Smith apples, cut into small chunks

- 1 ½ tablespoon and ½ teaspoon creamy salad dressing

- ⅔ cup chopped walnuts, or to taste

- 1 stalks celery, chopped

- 1 tablespoon lemon juice

- 2 ½ tablespoons and ½ teaspoon vanilla yogurt

- 1 ⅓ cooked chicken breasts, shredded

- 1 red onion, chopped

- 8 ⅓ seedless red grapes, halved

Instructions

1.   Combine the apple chunks, red onion, walnuts, shredded chicken, celery, and lemon juice in a large mixing bowl.

2.   Combine the vanilla yogurt, salad dressing, and mayonnaise; pour over the chicken mix and swirl to coat.

3.   Toss fresh grapes into the mix gently.

Nutrition Facts

Fat 22.7g; Protein 17.7g; Sodium 127.5mg

Chapter 7: Dinner Recipes For Intermittent Fasting

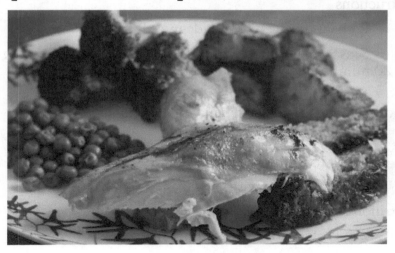

7.1 Honey Sesame Salmon

Prep Time: 20 minutes
Cook Time: 20 minutes
Servings: 2
Ingredients

- Pepper, for sprinkling

- Salt, for sprinkling

- 1-pound salmon fillets

- 1/4 cup water

- 2 tablespoons of sesame oil

- 1/4 cup honey

- 2 tablespoons of soy sauce

- 2 cloves garlic, crushed

- juice of 1 lemon

- 1/2 teaspoon Cornstarch, dissolved.

Instructions

1. Preheat the oven to 375 degrees F.

2. Season the salmon with salt and pepper before baking it for 20 minutes (cook time will depend on fillet size).

3. Meanwhile, add water, lemon, honey, sesame oil, soy sauce, and garlic to a saucepan.

4. Bring the water to a boil.

5. Cook until the cornstarch mixture has thickened.

6. Serve the sauce with the fish.

Nutrition Facts

Fat 13.2 g; Protein 31.7 g; Sodium 446.7 mg

7.2 Chicken with Cauliflower Rice Casserole

Prep Time: 60 minutes
Cook Time: 25 minutes
Servings: 2

Ingredients

- 3 cups shredded cooked chicken breast

- ¼ teaspoon cayenne pepper

- 2 teaspoons garlic powder

- ½ teaspoon ground pepper

- 6 ounces' cream cheese, softened

- ¼ teaspoon salt

- 1 (12-ounce) package of riced cauliflower

- ½ cup scallions

- 1 teaspoon dry mustard

- 1 teaspoon dried oregano

- 1 teaspoon onion powder

- 1 ½ cups shredded Cheddar cheese

Instructions

1.   Preheat the oven to 400 degrees Fahrenheit.

2.   Using cooking spray, cover a baking dish.

3.   In a microwave-safe bowl, place the cauliflower. Cover closely and heat on high for 4 minutes, or until tender.

4.   In a large mixing bowl, combine garlic powder, cream cheese, oregano, mustard, pepper, onion powder, salt, cayenne, and 14 cup scallions; mix with an electric blender on medium speed 1 minute, or until smooth.

5.   Combine the cauliflower, chicken, and 1 cup of Cheddar cheese in a mixing bowl.

6.   Fill the baking dish halfway with the mixture. Cover with foil and top with the remaining 12 cups of Cheddar.

7.   Bake for 30 minutes or until bubbling. Uncover and bake for another 10 minutes, or until the cheese is golden brown.

8.   Remove the pan from the oven and top with the remaining 14 cup scallions.

9.   Allow for a 10-minute rest period before serving.

Nutrition Facts

Fat 13g; Protein 32g; Sodium 439mg;

7.3 Lentil and Vegetable Curry

Prep Time: 60 minutes
Cook Time: 25 minutes
Servings: 2
Ingredients

- 300g (1 small) eggplant, cut into 2.5cm dice

- 1 tablespoon olive oil

- 3/4 cup dried French-style lentils

- 1 large onion, thinly sliced

- 400g (1/2 medium) cauliflower, cut into small florets

- 1/2 cup reduced-fat plain yogurt, to serve

- 1/2 reduced-salt vegetable stock cube, crumbled

- 150g green beans, topped, halved

- 400g can no added salt chopped tomatoes

- 2 tablespoons korma paste

- 100g button mushrooms, halved

- 2 garlic cloves, crushed

- 1/2 cup chopped coriander

- 2 1/2 cups of water

- 2 small whole meal pita bread, halved, to serve

Instructions

1.　　Heat the oil in a big, deep nonstick frying pan or a large deep saucepan at medium heat. Cook, often tossing, for 3-4 minutes, or when the onion and garlic you've added are tender and light golden in color.

2.　　Combine the korma paste and lentils in a mixing bowl. Cook for 1 minute, stirring constantly. Add the tomatoes, water, and stock cube to a mixing bowl. Put the water to a boil. Lower the heat, cover with the lid and cook for 10 minutes.

3.　　Combine the cauliflower, eggplant, and mushrooms in a bowl and mix. Cook for 15 minutes with the lid on. Add the beans and mix well. Simmer for another 5 minutes, uncovered, or until veggies are soft. Remove the pan from the heat. Add the coriander and mix well.

4.　　Serve with pita bread and yogurt.

Nutrition Facts

Fat 4.2g; Protein 6.2g; Sodium 416mg;

7.4 Honey Garlic Shrimp

Prep Time: 15 minutes
Cook Time: 5 minutes
Servings: 4

Ingredients

- 1 lb. medium shrimp
- 1/4 cup of soy sauce
- 3 teaspoons olive oil
- chopped green onion
- 1/3 cup of honey
- 2 garlic cloves, crushed
- 1 teaspoon minced ginger

Instructions

1.   Combine the honey, soy sauce, garlic, and ginger in a medium mixing bowl. Half will be used for the marinade,

and the other half will be used to cook the shrimp.

2.   Put the shrimp in a big sealable container or a bag. Pour half of the marinade/sauce mixture on top, give it a good shake or mix, and let the shrimp marinate for 15 minutes or up to 8 hours in the refrigerator. The rest of the marinade should be covered and kept refrigerated.

3.   In a pan, heat the olive oil over medium-high heat. In a skillet, place the shrimp. (Remove the used marinade.) Cook for 45 seconds on one side, then flip to cook for another 45 seconds. Pour in the remaining marinade/sauce and simmer until the shrimp is fully cooked, approximately 1-2 minutes longer.

4.   Serve the shrimp with the prepared marinade sauce and a green onion garnish on brown rice with steamed veggies on the side.

7.5 Turkey Meatball and Kale Soup

Prep Time: 5 minutes
Cook Time: 15 minutes
Servings: 2

Ingredients

- 1/2 lb. ground turkey

- Olive oil

- Bone broth for the soup

- 1 flax egg

- 1/4 cup almond flour

Instructions

1. In a medium mixing bowl, combine all of the ingredients and add season to taste.

2. Sear in olive oil in a medium saucepan, but don't cook all the way through. When the meat is boiling in the broth, it will continue to cook.

3. Cook with minced garlic, salt and pepper, red pepper flakes, and Italian seasoning in your favorite bone broth.

4. Add the carrots, 2 handfuls of chopped kale, and the turkey meatballs after the liquid has reached a steady boil.

5. Reduce heat to low and cook for 10 minutes. And then serve.

Nutrition Facts

Fat 6.0g; Protein 14.8g; Sodium 110.2mg

7.6 Chicken Provolone

Prep Time: 5 minutes
Cook Time: 25 minutes
Servings: 4

Ingredients

- 4 slices provolone cheese

- 1/4 teaspoon pepper

- 4 thin slices prosciutto or deli ham

- Butter-flavored cooking spray

- 8 fresh basil leaves

- 4 boneless skinless chicken breast halves (4 ounces each)

Instructions

1.   Season the chicken with salt and pepper.

2.   Cook chicken in a large pan sprayed with cooking spray until the thermometer reaches 165°, about 4-5 minutes on each side.

3.   Top with basil, prosciutto, and cheese on an ungreased ba king sheet.

4.   Broil 6-8 inches from the flame for 1-2 minutes, or until cheese is melted.

Nutrition Facts

Fat 6g; Protein 33g; Sodium 435mg

7.7 Spaghetti Diablo with Shrimp

Prep Time: 5 minutes
Cook Time: 25 minutes
Servings: 4
Ingredients

- ½ teaspoon olive oil

- ½ onion, chopped

- 1 can of diced tomatoes

- ¼ cup white wine

- 6 ounces cooked shrimp

- salt and ground black pepper

- ½ green bell pepper, chopped

- ¼ cup grated Pecorino-Romano cheese

- ½ yellow bell pepper, chopped

- 4 ounces' spaghetti

- ¼ teaspoon dried oregano

- 3 cloves garlic, crushed

- ¼ teaspoon red pepper flakes

- ¼ cup chopped fresh parsley, divided

- ¼ teaspoon dried basil

Instructions

1.   In a Dutch oven, heat the oil over medium-high heat. 5 to 7 minutes in heated oil, stir and cook yellow bell pepper, green bell pepper, onions, and garlic until soft.

2.   Season with salt & pepper.

3.   Bring the bell pepper combination to a boil with the tomatoes, alcohol, 1/4 cup parsley, oregano, basil and red pepper flakes; lower heat to low and cover the Dutch oven.

4.   Cook, stirring regularly, for approximately 2 hours, or until the tomatoes have broken down.

5.   Bring a big saucepan of water to a boil, lightly salted. Cook spaghetti in boiling water for approximately 10 minutes.

6.   Cook, occasionally stirring, until the drained pasta and shrimp are fully cooked but still stiff to the touch, 2 to 4 minutes longer.

7.   Toss with the remaining Pecorino-Romano cheese and parsley before serving.

Nutrition Facts

Fat 3.5g; Protein 29g; Sodium 233mg

Chapter 8: Dessert Recipes For Intermittent Fasting

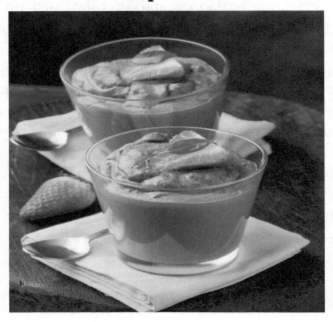

8.1 Citrus Dark Chocolate Mousse

Prep Time: 5 minutes
Cook Time: 15 minutes
Servings: 5

Ingredients

- 1 tsp of brewed coffee

- 85g of dark chocolate

- 1 pinch of rock salt

- 1 tsp of orange zest

- 1/2 tsp of lime zest

- 3 medium eggs

Instructions

1.   In a small dish, combine orange and lime zest.

2.   On top of the double boiler, combine the chocolate and coffee with the zest over warm water.

3.   To keep the mixture from bubbling, stir it.

4.   Remove the chocolate from the heat after it has melted and set it aside to cool.

5.   The egg whites and salt should be whisked together.

6.   Stir the egg yolks in the chocolate mixture, then pour the mixture over the egg whites and gently fold them in.

7.   Make small bowls or glasses out of the mixture. Refrigerate for at least 4 hours before serving.

Nutrition Facts

Fat 36g; Protein 10g; Sodium 294mg;

8.2 Peanut Butter Cookies

Prep Time: 15 minutes
Cook Time: 10 minutes
Servings: 24

Ingredients

- ½ teaspoon salt

- 2 large eggs

- 1 ½ teaspoons baking soda

- 1 cup crunchy peanut butter

- 1 cup unsalted butter

- 1 teaspoon baking powder

- 1 cup white sugar

- 2 ½ cups all-purpose flour

- 1 cup packed brown sugar

Instructions

1.   In a mixing bowl, combine together cream butter, peanut butter, and sugar; add in the eggs.

2.   Mix flour, baking powder, baking soda, and salt in a separate dish, then add the butter mixture. Refrigerate the dough for 1 hour.

3.   Make 1 inch balls out of the dough and place them on baking pans. Using a fork, flatten each ball into a crisscross pattern. Bake for approximately 10 minutes in a preheated 375°F oven until the cookies appear brown.

Nutrition Facts

Fat 136g; Protein 4.5g; Sodium 209.4mg;

8.3 Fruit Salad

Prep Time: 5 minutes
Cook Time: 20 minutes
Servings: 8

Ingredients

- 4 kiwis

- 1 cocktail strawberries

- 20 ounces of can pineapple chunks

- 2 apples

- 2 bananas

- 1 can of peach pie filling

Instructions

1.   Toss the diced apples with the leftover pineapple juice in a small bowl. Allow resting for 7 to 10 minutes.

2.   Combine the peach pie and pineapple pieces in a large salad dish.

3.   Remove the apples from the pineapple juice and combine them with the pie filling and pineapple mixture in a mixing bowl. Let 7 to 10 minutes for the sliced bananas to soak up the saved pineapple juice.

4.   Peel and slice the kiwifruit, as well as half of the strawberries. Set aside the remaining half of the strawberries.

5.   Remove the bananas from the pineapple juice and stir them into the pie filling. Toss in the strawberries that have been cut.

6.   Arrange kiwi slices and strawberry slices around the edges of the serving basin. Chill before serving.

Nutrition Facts

Fat 0.5g; Protein 2.1g; Sodium 15mg;

8.1 Grapefruit Meringue Nests with Mixed Berries

Prep Time: 25 minutes
Cook Time: 1 hour 30 minutes
Servings: 8

Ingredients

Meringue Nests

- 1 teaspoon grapefruit peel

- 1/2 cup sugar

- 4 egg whites

- 1/8 teaspoon cream of tartar

Berries

- 4 ounces of raspberries

- ¼ cup sugar

- 2 lbs. strawberries

- 4 ounces of blueberries

- ¼ cup of grapefruit juice

Instructions

Meringues

1.   Preheat the oven to 200 °F.

2.   Use parchment paper to line a large cookie sheet.

3.   In a large mixer, mix egg whites and cream.

4.   Sprinkle in sugar 2 tbsp, beating until sugar dissolves, and meringue stands in stiff, creamy peaks.

5.   Gently mix grapefruit peel into a meringue.

6.   On a prepared sheet, divide the mixture into even mounds and spaced approximately 3 inches apart.

7.   Form mounds into 3-inch circular nests by pressing the back of a spoon into the center of each meringue.

8.   Bake for 2 hours until firm.

9.   Turn off the oven and let the meringues in there to dry for 2 hours or overnight.

10.   Remove the parchment gently after it has dried.

11.   Meringues may be kept at room temperature for up to 2 weeks.

Berries

1.   Combine blueberries, raspberries, and half of the strawberries in a large mixing bowl.

2.   Add sugar and grapefruit juice to a 12-inch skillet.

3.   On medium heat to boiling, stir now and then

4.   Boil for 2 minutes, or until the sugar has dissolved and the syrup has turned a clear pink color.

5.   Cook for 1-3 minutes, or until the first half of the strawberries have released their juices and softened.

6.   In a large mixing basin, pour the mixture over the uncooked berries.

7.   Stir slowly until everything is fully blended.

8. Place the nests of meringue on serving plates.

9. Spread berries among the nests and sprinkle with grapefruit syrup.

10. Serve right away.

Nutrition Facts

Fat 40g; Protein 20g; Sodium 400mg;

8.5 Mango and Passionfruit Roulade

Prep Time: 20 minutes
Cook Time: 15 minutes
Servings: 4

Ingredients

- 85g of sugar

- 3 eggs

- 250g of frozen raspberries

- 1 tsp of vanilla extract

- One tub of Greek yogurt

- 2 mangoes

- 85g plain flour, sifted

- 1 tsp baking powder

- 1 tbsp of sugar

- 2 ripe passion fruits

Instructions

1. Preheat the oven to 180°C.

2. In a large mixing bowl, mix the eggs and sugar until it's thick and light. After that, fold in the flour and baking powder, followed by the vanilla.

3.   Place the mixture in the pan, tilting it to level it out, and bake for 14-15 minutes until it's brown. Place on a new piece of paper that has been powdered with 1 tbsp caster sugar. Allow cooling fully after rolling the paper within the sponge.

4.   Fold the sugar, passion fruit pulp, and one-third of the mango and raspberries. Unroll the sponge, spread with filling, then roll-up.

Nutrition Facts

Fat 3g; Protein 5g; Sodium 256mg;

8.6 Strawberry-Chocolate Greek Yogurt

Prep Time: 10 minutes
Cook Time: 180 minutes
Servings: 32
Ingredients

- 1 cup of sliced strawberries

- 2 tbsp. of honey

- ¼ cup of chocolate chips

- 3 cups plain Greek yogurt

- 1 teaspoon vanilla extract

Instructions

1.   Using parchment paper, line in a baking sheet.

2.   Combine the yogurt, honey, and vanilla extract in a medium mixing bowl.

3.   Make a rectangle on the lined baking sheet.

4.   Sprinkle the chocolate chips on top and spread the strawberries on top.

5.   Freeze for at least 3 hours, or until extremely firm. Cut to pieces to serve.

Nutrition Facts

Fat 1.3g; Protein 2g; Sodium 7.6mg

8.7 Almond Butter Chocolate Chip Cookies

Prep Time: 15 minutes
Cook Time: 35 minutes
Servings: 15

Ingredients

- ¼ cup chopped peanuts

- 1 egg

- 1 cup of almond butter

- ½ cup of chocolate chips

- 1 teaspoon of baking soda

- ½ cup of brown sugar

Instructions

1. Preheat the oven to 350°F. Line two baking pans with parchment paper.

2. In a medium mixing bowl, whisk together the egg.

3. Combine almond butter, brown sugar, and baking soda in a mixing bowl and whisk until smooth.

4. Combine peanuts and chocolate chips in a mixing bowl.

5. To create each cookie, take roughly 1 tablespoon of dough and roll it into a compact ball.

6. Place the cookies 1 inch apart on the prepared pan pans. With the tip of a spoon, gently push down on each ball.

7. Bake the cookies for 9 to 10 minutes, or until the tops are cracked, and the edges are brown.

8. Allow cooling for 10 minutes on the pan.

Nutrition Facts

Fat 10g; Protein 4g; Sodium 108mg

Conclusion

In conclusion, intermittent fasting has indeed been scientifically proven to be a pleasant and effective way to lose weight and get favorable health advantages for women over 60. Intermittent fasting is a method of allowing the body to metabolize the food it has consumed. On the other hand, scientists have discovered that this fasting approach is not suited for everyone. As a result, it's a good idea to get medical advice before fasting. Intermittent fasting side effects are caused by the body's inability to adjust to the new eating schedule. As one continues to fast, the body will get used to it, and the negative effects will disappear. Intermittent fasting should also be avoided if one has a history of health problems, such as high blood pressure. Intermittent fasting is a fantastic alternative to difficult-to-maintain fad diets for women over 60. Time-restricted eating allows women to lose weight without limiting their calorie intake or depriving themselves of essential nutrients. Intermittent fasting may easily be incorporated into everyday activities as part of a well-balanced diet. It is a kind of eating that alternates between eating and fasting intervals. Intermittent fasting may be done in a variety of ways, including twice-weekly, alternate-day, and time-restricted.

Intermittent fasting has various effects on women. Women should be aware of potential dangers to their reproductive health, bone health, and general well-being. Whereas with disadvantages, there are certain advantages like weight reduction, diabetes prevention, and improved heart health are all potential health advantages of intermittent fasting, according to evidence.

While fasting, understanding how one reacts to various meals might assist in eating in a beneficial manner for metabolic health. There are a few things one can do to maximize the health advantages of intermittent fasting. Using a notebook to keep track of the routine may help to notice improvement and motivate one to exercise, prevent snacking, and eat at the right times. It may also urge one to develop a fasting habit or lifestyle.

When fasting, it's also beneficial to remain aware. Take time to exercise and re-energize the body to remain active and on track with one's dietary cycles. This may help one to get the most out of the workouts, avoid weight gain, and keep track of the food intake.

Making an intermittent fasting schedule will assist in being active and adhering to a fasting lifestyle. It has a plethora of health advantages that may last a lifetime. If fasting is safe for you, it is well worth it to gain the many health advantages of intermittent fasting.

Made in United States
Troutdale, OR
10/10/2023

13573950R00050